SEX GUIDE FOR WOMEN

SECRETS TO BETTER YOUR SEX LIFE NOW

OLIVIA HAWCK

CONTENTS

Sensual Massage	1
The Erogenous Zones	4
Sensual Massage in Sex Therapy	7
How Is a Sensual Massage	9
Beginners Guide to Sensual Massage	11
Gels and Oils Used for Sensual Massage	14
Sensual Massage Techniques	16
Advanced Sensual Massage	19

©Copyright 2022 by Olivia Hawck
All rights Reserved

ISBN: 978-1-63970-119-3

In no way is it legal to reproduce, duplicate, or transmit any part of this document in either electronic means or in printed format. Recording of this publication is strictly prohibited and any storage of this document is not allowed unless with written permission from the publisher. All rights are reserved.
Respective authors own all copyrights not held by the publisher.

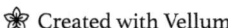 Created with Vellum

SENSUAL MASSAGE

*M*assage is direct stimulation of the outer and inner layers of the muscles and tissues of the body using different techniques. It helps in the healing of the tissues and develops a sense of well-being and relaxation. The term 'massage' is directly borrowed from the French word massage, and an examination of the word's root around the globe (Arabic 'massa', Greek 'masso', Latin 'massa') would reveal that the term means dough or knead and you get to see a lot of kneading movements in massage.

Massage involves the movement of hands or different parts of the body or a mechanical tool over the body at various degrees of pressure, movements, tension, or vibration on another body. It can benefit the whole body or part of it or various internal organs.

Over the years, massages have gained the reputation of being a cure for many ailments and as a lifestyle for many around the globe.

Sensual massage is a pleasurable variation of this technique in which the body's erogenous zones are massaged. This helps in arousal and even enhancing sexual performance and health.

This is not anything new, as the health benefits of sexual or sensual massage have been known and practiced for a long time. While the main area of focus in sensual massage for males is the genital area, it also includes their breasts for women. Genital massage may also be termed mutual masturbation.

Nowadays, this is a part of therapy, foreplay, or even post-sex.

Sensual Massage, unlike Traditional Massage, appeals to all senses. This is what makes it unique, and this is what needs to be noted.

We have five senses
a.The eyes
b.The ears
c.The nose
d.The palate
e.The skin

IN TRADITIONAL MASSAGE, only the skin is tended to. However, as the other sense is also to be taken care of in Sensual Massage, there needs to be a preparations procedure.

The ambiance is of prime importance. This will take care of three senses by itself.

The room should be warm to the feel and the sight. A fireplace is the best place to indulge in a Sensual Massage or a warm-colored room with red or orange paint or curtains. The light should primarily come from candles, or the electrical bulbs downed to a dim shimmer.

You can use scented candles and ambergris or incense sticks that are not overpowering and don't smoke the room. A light and soft music played at a soft volume also adds to the body and mind's relaxation. The eyes, nose, and eras are tended to at just the ambiance alone.

Food also plays a significant part in Sensual Massage. It may range from sweet red wine to dry fruits or dates and grapes. Some people also take elaborate courses like spicy roasted meat and bread in small portions. If you use spicy foods, remember to clean your mouth and hands completely with mild soap.

Unlike Traditional Massage, you are not limited to any part of the body, and you can touch the intimate parts. But be sure that your partner enjoys your touch. It is more about giving than receiving, so make it a point to let your partner know that you would like to provide something special. It is also good to leave the room while your partner gets undressed and have a sheet to cover themselves with. Never rush anything, and it's good to not have an aim when indulging in a Sensual Massage.

Sensual Massage is a good way to build trust among partners and deepen the bonds you already have. It makes you feel better in your intimate moments and also understand true relationships. It takes lovemaking to a level that you make 'love' and bring on newer meanings to your intimate relations. Some exercises even let you feel connected so deep that you feel as if your souls are connected. It also lets you feel less ashamed and also revel in your nudity in front of your partner.

THE EROGENOUS ZONES

The term is taken from the Greek Eros, meaning love, and Genes meaning born. Therefore, the term applies to any part of the body that has a level of sensitivity at a heightened level as there are several nerve endings. The stimulation of these parts directly or indirectly produces sexual arousal, fantasies, and even orgasm.

Erogenous zones are spread all over the body. Some areas are more sensitive than others. Depending on the body, stimulation of these parts can produce different levels of arousal. To give a sensual massage, a thorough understanding of the erogenous zones is essential as an immediate orgasm may often reduce the effects of the massage.

THE EROGENOUS ZONES **are divided into two categories:**

1. NONSPECIFIC ZONES: These areas resemble normal skin and have many nerve endings that help in heightened stimulation. The nape of the neck, inner arms, etc., are some examples.

2.Specific Zones: These areas are denser in nerve endings and often cause direct sexual arousal. It is said that they have a close connection with the brain and the brain's reward system.

For males, the focus falls on the pubic region mainly. The erogenous zones are the areas like the top part of the glans and the sides, the side of the penis, the scrotum, the perineum, the anus and the surrounding areas.

There are many more erogenous zones when it comes to women.

The genital area of women is called the vulva. The clitoris and the outer parts of the vagina have many nerve endings and can be stimulated even to reach an orgasm without penetration.

OTHER EROGENOUS AREAS INCLUDE:

1.THE SCALP: A massage to the scalp or a caress of the hair is relaxing yet stimulating to many.

2.The nape of the neck is a very sensitive part and is usually aroused by kissing, biting (softly), or licking. It is a susceptible zone in females and the place where 'love bites' are found.

3.The Ear: The outer sides of the ear and the lobe are sensitive areas that respond to licking or nibbling.

4.The Chest: The entire breast area of both men and women has several nerve endings and can be aroused using the hands. The areola and the nipples are also highly sensitive. Stimulating the hair around the areola produces oxytocin and directly stimulates the genital region.

5.The Abdomen: The lower part of the abdomen and the entire navel is very responsive to touch. They also bring about stimulation to the genital areas primarily due to their proximity.

6.The Arms: The softer inner parts of the arm and the end of the arm are incredibly erogenous to both men and women.

7.The Armpits: This is a highly erogenous area, especially if it has hair on it. Slowly caressing the armpit is a very stimulating experience, and it is also believed to produce pheromones in men and women.

8.The Fingers: The fingers, especially the tips and the top cone, have an abundance of nerve endings and can be stimulated orally.

9.The Legs: The inner part of the thighs leading to the pubic region is a very responsive one to caresses and light massages.

10.The Feet: Especially the toes as there are many nerve endings, responds to caresses and oral stimulation. The rough areas at the knees and ankles are also found to create an erogenous sensation if stimulated with soft caresses.

SENSUAL MASSAGE IN SEX THERAPY

Sensual Massage plays an important role in Sex Therapy these days. This has manifold effects on the sexual well-being, but it is mainly used to stimulate and enhance their libido (positive response to sexual stimuli. It is also done by professionals on men who have premature ejaculation issues.

The use of Sensual Genital Massage has reference to being used by physicians to treat women having Female Hysteria. This was popular as a treatment until finally, the patients were referred to midwives. However, it was time-consuming, and the patients needed treatment regularly.

Some techniques have been derived from research that enhances orgasm in both men and women. One such method is called Extended Orgasm. It does not come under normal orgasms but can be explained as much more intense sensations that last anywhere from minutes to an hour or more. In addition, the orgasms have been reported to have reached a full-body level.

Some reports also show that contractions and energetic stimulation are seen all around the body, mainly at the abdomen, genitals, hands, and inner thighs. There have also been different states of consciousness connected with the orgasm bordering on the spiritual level, as explained in the Tantric Sex Texts.

NEO TANTRA

This is the Western modification of Tantric Sex. Tantric Sex elevates sexual satisfaction to a spiritual level, whereas the former is not that much into the spiritual level attainment. The Western Neo-Tantra has come to be after thorough research on the Buddhist and Hindu Tantra.

It involves all the rituals of the traditional one and has brought forth many unorthodox movements. There is also a famous school of thought called Sex Magic.

HOW IS A SENSUAL MASSAGE

*S*ensual Massage can be done alone or with a partner. It can be used for various reasons, the main ones being:
1. Reaching or enhancing orgasms
2. A heightened level of foreplay

CONTROLLED ORGASMS

Controlled orgasms heighten the level of sexual release to a heightened level and even may never stimulate levels of consciousness. This can be done alone or with the help of a partner. It is a technique of maintaining the highest level of arousal for extended periods. Although the climax plateau of men is lower than that of women, using this technique, men can go for repeated coitus without the delay of refractory periods that come after regular orgasms. It is a series of peaked sexual stimuli without a complete release of sexual tension. When the final release is made, the orgasm attained is so high that it results in multiple orgasms and states of mind called Euphoric.

. . .

ORGASM CONTROL WITH A PARTNER

This is a sex game that involves sensual massage as the foreplay, building up the tension, and giving complete control of the orgasm to the partner. The receiver is made to reach the stimulation level just below that orgasm's Point of No Return. This is done by altering the speed and stimulation of the sexual activity involved. This is done multiple times by giving small gaps that bring the heightened tension level to almost zero. All the tensions that have been 'denied' build-up, and the final orgasm(s) will be much heightened.

MASTURBATION:

This is practiced to attain higher levels of orgasmic release or to prolong the coitus with a partner. People usually follow a masturbation 'exercise' as they are in full control of regulating their peaks and troughs of sexual tension. There are two ways of attaining this.

1. Edging: This is done by letting go of all stimulation just before sexual release and letting the stimulated tension go all the way to zero, and building it up again.

2. Surfing: In this variation, there is no complete letting go but continue with the stimulation at a reduced level of intensity.

BEGINNERS GUIDE TO SENSUAL MASSAGE

Now that you know the benefits and techniques involved in Sensual Massage, let's look at how to give it to your partner:

TOOLKIT:

1. A Massage Bed: Since it will involve many sexual stimulation and gaps that reduce tension, it is best to give the message to your partner on a bed. A bed at the proper height will also be easy on your back as you will not have to strain your pose or muscles.

2. A Pillow: Your partner must shift from a prone position to a flat on back position. When your partner takes a horizontal position, a pillow under the knees is very relaxing, and when lying flat on the tummy, a pillow under the head is to be offered.

3. Thick Blanket: If you offer massage in a setting like a fireplace or don't have a massage bed, a blanket will come in handy.

4. Scented candles and incense sticks also create an ambiance that gets all the cozier with a soft music playing in the background.

5. Last but not least, a selection of lubricants. Though you can give a sensual massage with a base oil, it is much better to use an Aromatherapy oil. Some also have an aphrodisiac effect but pay close attention to the dilution of the Aromatherapy Oils as some may be harmful and cause allergic reactions.

THE BASICS:

1. Arrange a cozily warm room. A massage is no going to be a good experience for a person they are cold. Slow music, reduced lighting, and some fragrances will set the complete mood for you.

2. Let them feel that you are offering something special as a token of love.

3. Always start with lying flat on the back with their head resting on a pillow or a folded blanket. This is done so that there is no direct stimulation to the genitals at the start and build up the mood. People are less shy to start with a back massage than a frontal one.

4. Apply a little bit of warm oil in your hands and start by massaging their back. Slow unbroken kneads or circles will do the job to warm up their mood.

5. The order of a massage is:
a. Back
b. Legs
c. Turnover and massage the feet
d. Legs
e. Arms
f. Shoulder
g. Scalp
h. Breasts and pubic region

6. You should not have a fixed schedule as 2 minutes to each part or so. If your partner wants a certain area to be massaged

more than just be in the giving mood. They eventually will be in the mood for a much intense massage.

NURU MASSAGE:

This Japanese form of massage tops the list as it is done body to body. It creates more closeness among partners as the massage is not done with the hands but with the whole body and makes a lot of intimacy and heightened levels of sexual stimulation.

Nuru means 'Slippery' and, contrary to the general rule in massage, 'not to overdo the lubricant.' This uses a generous amount on the body, and there are also special gels in the market.

This massage is done in the nude, i.e., both the partners are naked, and the closest you can get to penetration intimacy is present.

Start by applying the gel on your body, allowing a teasing glance to your partner and stimulating yourself. Pour a generous helping of the gel and use it on your partner with your hands first. Then massage their muscles with your forearms. Next, go side by side and continue with the sliding motion and mount on your partner. You can use your buttocks and groin area to massage them before going completely body to body. The best part of a Nuru Massage is that you can take turns in the same session.

GELS AND OILS USED FOR SENSUAL MASSAGE

Though there are many Aromatherapy Oils in the market, they are not solely for sensual Massages, so here are some other gels and oils that you can use.

1.Honey: Honey has many health benefits and about 190 nutrients that are nourishing for the body and detoxifying. It can be directly applied to wounds and gashes. It is also considered to be an aphrodisiac, and you can use your mouth or tongue to massage those unique places of your partner.

2.Lavender: This soothes the muscles and completely relaxes your partner. Inhaling the fumes of this oil also relaxes the mind and opens up your partner's mood for a sexual massage.

3.Aloe Vera: If you want to infuse many healthy benefits in your Sensual Massage, then Aloe Vera would come in the top list. It contains over 200 nourishing ingredients and is antibiotic and antifungal, to name a few benefits.

4.Orange Oil: This helps in blood circulation in the body and is especially stimulating if applied at Erogenous Zones of the body.

5.Peppermint: Mint and menthol have been long related to

sexual activity. The smallest suggestion of it will heighten the mood. It also relaxes the muscles

6.Rosemary: Rosemary is a muscle relaxant and best to use if your partner is tired or just not at his best.

7.Melilot: Melilot is also an effective relaxant and can relax your partner's mood.

SENSUAL MASSAGE TECHNIQUES

FOR MEN:
1. Begin with the head. All men love when their head is massaged. Start at the scalp and go down the head in soft circular motions.

2. Use a blend of oil that is known for its relaxing aroma, like Sandalwood.

3. Take a liberal helping of oil. It is best to patch test the oil if you have an Essential Oil kit, as some may cause allergic reactions.

4. Move slowly down from the head to the neck and then to the shoulder and the back.

5. Listen to feedback from him; if he wants a bit more attention at a specific spot, linger there a bit longer. Men usually love long caresses to the head.

6. Massage downwards as this is good for improving blood circulation. Use the type of pressure he likes (evident in his feedback). There are no hard and fast rules in Sensual Massage.

7. There are chances that he falls asleep. That is normal.

If you wish to wake him, do so after 20-25 minutes. Then, he will have had a very refreshing sleep and will feel rejuvenated.

TRIGGER ZONES IN MEN:

Paying particular attention to 'Trigger Zones' will heighten the efficiency of a sensual massage.

1.The Lips. The lower lip and its curve that leads down to the chin is a susceptible zone. Kissing his lip and using your tongue to caress it will make him come to his mood fast. This is especially good if he has fallen asleep and you need to wake him up after the 20 minutes gap.

2.The Neck: Use a feather or a soft kiss to stimulate nerve endings behind his neck (nape). Continue the motion unbroken along his collar bone and under his Adam's apple.

3.The Nipples: A man's nipples are just as sensitive as women's, and newer studies show that they are more sensitive than women's. Licking on the areola and rolling his nipples with your tongue is very stimulating.

4.The Inner Thighs. These are very sensitive to touch as they join at the pubic area. Slow circular motions at the inner thigh and a spreading motion that goes upward and back again with a random caress at the perineum is a sure tease for any man.

FOR WOMEN:

1.Start with moderate pressure on the lower back, avoid the spine, and work up in a gentle elliptical round spanning all her back.

2.Use your thumbs at the shoulders, massaging away any knots if you notice them. Always use slow pressure on the shoulders.

3.Go down her arm and massage her palms, rolling each finger slowly between your palms.

4.Women love foot massages, and paying particular attention

can make you a winner if she finds it tickly to go slower with a bit more pressure.

5. Listen for feedback moans or non-verbal signs like her body rising for contact with yours.

6. Gliding movements on her sides with a slow teasing touch at the sides of her breast are very stimulating as these are soft and sensitive areas.

7. When massaging her lying flat on her tummy, make slow inward motions at her inner thighs up to just under her pubic area and then down.

8. Make her roll over and massage her feet and legs. She will feel relaxed and open for many intimate touches.

ADVANCED SENSUAL MASSAGE

Once you have done some essential massages to your partner and become a regular thing in your love life, then it's time to go into advanced mode. Discuss it with your partner before going into this mode.

YONI MASSAGE

1. Yoni Massage: Yoni is the Sanskrit term for Vagina. This adds a spiritual twist to the massage and is about respecting her sacredness through reverence to her genitalia.

The woman lies on her back with pillows at her head and buttocks. Her legs are spread comfortably, and her Yoni in full view. Her partner sits directly in front and between her legs. Inhale through your nose and exhale from your mouth. The body is let to shed out negativity as each part is relaxed. She is starting at the head and going all the way down to the legs. Each breath relaxes each part of the body.

Apply a bit of oil to your palms and softly massage the inner thighs with alternating long and short and varied pressure up and down her inner thighs. Softly caress the Yoni in an up and down motion at first and then spreading the lips a bit. Pay attention to the outer folds of her Yoni, and once in her Yoni, look for feedback signs of what sensations she loves best. Apply a bit more oil before proceeding to her clitoris. Alternate touches and pressure and try softly pressing it with your fingers.

Yoni Massage is not focused on orgasm but an intimate bond between you and her. Prolong the session as long as she wants it to. Get to know her limit of arousal. If she reaches an orgasm, hug her as close and warm as possible and enjoy the feeling of your heart reflecting on the massage. You must maintain eye contact throughout the massage.

PROSTATE MASSAGE

1.Prostate Massage: This is commonly done on men. The prostate is the area surrounding his bladder and urethra. It is usually stimulated through the anus as it can be found near the anterior part of the rectum.

The person needs to empty his bowels, wash the anus with warm water and soap, and clean it more profound than usual. This is done with fingers and surgical gloves, and a lot of lubricants are advised. Never use your fingers directly as they can tear the soft tissues in the rectum.

Have him lie flat on a bed with his buttocks in a clear view. After he takes some deep breath and feels relaxed, inserts your finger slowly and deep until you reach a knot in the tunnel.

Use slow circular motions. Slowly increase the pressure and decrease it if he feels any discomfort. Some men become intensely aroused, but a prostate massage is done best if kept to 15 minutes or until he asks to stop.

Never make Prostate Massage a routine as it can lead to

severe medical conditions. Once in two weeks is the best to engage in it.

The End.

www.ingramcontent.com/pod-product-compliance
Lightning Source LLC
LaVergne TN
LVHW021750060526
838200LV00052B/3569